DR ALAN JASON

WHAT EXPERTS ARE SAYING ABOUT DIABETES

REVEALED SECRETS ABOUT DIABETES

Table of Contents

INTRODUCTION

Assuming you have diabetes, your body can't interact as expected and use glucose from the food you eat. There are various kinds of diabetes, each with various causes, yet they all offer the normal issue of having a lot of glucose in your circulation system. Medicines incorporate drugs as well as insulins. A few sorts of diabetes can be forestalled by embracing a solid way of life.

Diabetes happens when your body can't take up sugar (glucose) into its cells and use it for energy. This results in a development of additional sugar in your circulatory system.

Inadequately controlled diabetes can prompt serious outcomes, causing harm to a large number of your body's organs and tissues, including your heart, kidneys, eyes and nerves. Diabetes side effects rely heavily on how high your glucose is. Certain individuals, particularly assuming they have prediabetes or type 2 diabetes, might not have side effects. In type 1 diabetes, side effects will generally come on rapidly and be more extreme.

Chapter 1: Diabetes:

1.1 What Is It and Who Gets It?

Diabetes is a huge issue in the created world, and is particularly pervasive among specific ethnic gatherings. However many individuals are not quite certain what diabetes is, who gets it, and whether they are in danger. The Nuts and bolts Diabetes implies an excessive amount of sugar in the blood. Its appropriate name is diabetes mellitus.

The sugar in the diabetic individual's framework additionally turns out in the pee, which diabetics produce a ton of, the old Egyptians saw that the pee of specific individuals pulled in sugar-cherishing bugs like subterranean insects. The expression "diabetes" comes from the Greek doctor Arateus, and signifies "to siphon.

"The expression "mellitus" (signifying "honey sweet") occurred in the last part of the 1600s. Diabetics need to do whatever it takes to control their glucose levels, something typically done consequently inside the body. How this is finished and how much it is done relies upon the sort of diabetes that is available.

1.2 Types

There are two essential kinds of diabetes. Type1 diabetes, additionally called adolescent diabetes, frequently happens in youth. In this kind of diabetes, the pancreatic cells are obliterated, either by the body's own resistant framework or an outside harm to the pancreas, like injury or medical procedure. Type 1 diabetics should infuse insulin into their bodies since their pancreas no longer creates insulin. Insulin takes the sugar from the blood and gets it into the body's cells where it very well may be utilized.

Type II diabetes is undeniably more normal and will in general happen in grown-ups. For the most part, those with Type II diabetes have a working pancreas; it simply doesn't create sufficient insulin, or the insulin it produces is "overlooked" by the body (insulin obstruction). Type II diabetes can once in a while be dealt with diet and exercise, and insulin infusions could conceivably be important.

1.3 What Causes Diabetes?

Chances are, you know somebody with diabetes, or somebody in your family has it. Yet, what causes it? How does an individual foster the side effects of diabetes? There are fundamentally two sorts of diabetes, Type I and Type II. These contrast regarding their goal and treatment. Here are a few thoughts regarding what causes diabetes. Type I diabetes is brought about by a breaking down pancreas.

What makes the pancreas breakdown varies from one case to another. It will in general run in families, however a few people have diabetes in youth when nobody in their family has any set of experiences of the sickness. In certain people, their own resistant framework goes after the pancreas and annihilates its phones, subsequently delivering it futilely. In others with Type I diabetes, a physical issue or pancreatic medical procedure obliterates the pancreas to the point that it can never again create insulin. Type I diabetes has an unexpected segment in comparison to Type II. Kids really youthful determined to have Type I diabetes - thus the substitute name for Type I diabetes is adolescent diabetes. In any case, more seasoned individuals can surely foster Sort diabetes, particularly assuming there is injury to the pancreas. Type II diabetes might have a few genetic variables, as well, yet not to the obvious degree that Type I does. In Type II, the body becomes impervious to the insulin that the pancreas is yet delivering. Or on the other hand, Type II diabetics have a working pancreas yet the organ doesn't deliver sufficient insulin.

More established people and the individuals who are overweight are viewed as more in danger of creating Type II diabetes than those with a sound body weight and way of life. What Triggers It? An auto-safe confusion could set off Type I diabetes, as the body's resistant framework can mysteriously go after the pancreas and obliterate its cells. There could likewise be some alternate way that the pancreas gets harmed, which isn't age explicit. Type II diabetes might be set off by undesirable, sugar-rich eating regimens and a stationary way of life. The pancreas may just become depleted attempting to keep the glucose down in light of the steady deluge of sugar from the eating regimen.

Different opportunities for triggers incorporate hypertension and stress. While it's not straightforwardly demonstrated as a causal element, people with hypertension are genuinely bound to foster diabetes than those with typical pulse. Stress as a causal component has a correspondingly problematic status, yet frequently thought by clinical experts delayed, unrelieved pressure builds the gamble of diabetes. At times the pressure is brought about by injury or profound unsettling influence, some way or another making the individual vulnerable to creating diabetes.

1.4 Who Gets Diabetes?

Type I diabetes will in general spat families. Type II diabetes can likewise run in families, and may happen to people: the individuals who are overweight, stationary, beyond 35 years old, or had gestational diabetes before. You can't "get" diabetes as it isn't brought about by a microorganism. The predominant assessment among clinical experts is that Type II diabetes can be forestalled or limited through a solid way of life. The hypothesis goes that an excessive amount of white flour items, white sugar, corn syrup, and other refined sugars and grains make the pancreas become depleted or the body to oppose the insulin that is delivered.

Chapter 2: Diabetes in Kids - An Aide for Families

Has your kid been determined to have diabetes, and you're stressed? Or on the other hand perhaps the individual has had diabetes for some time yet you feel like you're struggling. At times, guardians and families need to comprehend what diabetes means for the relational peculiarity, and how they can be steady. Whether your kid is a baby, youngster, or in grade school, families frequently need some direction on how they can assist their youngsters with carrying on with a typical life. Here is a concise aide for families living with youngsters who have diabetes. Be Prepared for Misguided judgments Guardians and diabetic kids should manage different confusions and fantasies about diabetes. It's great to investigate a portion of the more common fantasies and questions, and have a prepared solution for them.

You might need to mentor your kid in noting these misinterpretations too:

"Will I get diabetes from you/your kid?" obviously not - diabetes isn't transferable.

"I can't welcome you/your kid to my birthday celebration!" Youngsters with diabetes may not be welcome to birthday celebrations on the grounds that many hosts/guardians don't need the obligation of a diabetic kid, particularly one encompassed by sweet birthday treats. Ideally, you can work with the guardians of children who are having birthday celebrations and let your kid partake in anything you're alright with.

"Will you pass on assuming you eat sugar?" Certain individuals feel that diabetics will be "harmed" assuming that they eat sugar.

"You probably ate an excess of sugar as a child/kid; that is the reason you have diabetes."

Many individuals imagine that eating a lot of sugar causes diabetes. Exploration To assist with causing the sickness to appear to be less unnerving, research the phrasing and real factors of the illness. Like that, when your primary care physician converses with you about the sickness, you won't feel scared by the terms and will understand what the individual in question is referring to. Information can assist you with feeling enabled.

You can likewise utilize your exploration to assist with concocting a strategy, which causes a ton of families to have a solid sense of reassurance. Incorporate Other Relatives When you can, remember the family for the booked feast times and even bites. A few families make a daily together season of the bite before bed that most diabetics need. Everybody in the family ought to know how to perceive indications of an issue, high or low glucose particularly.

2.0 Get Involved

Include yourself in the diabetes local area in your space and additionally on the web. There are diabetes camps, online structures, and different care groups that can assist your family with living with diabetes. These gatherings can likewise assist your youngster with figuring out how to adapt to diabetes now and later on.

Signs and Side effects of Diabetes in Babies, Kids and Grown-ups.

Diabetes isn't as extraordinary a sickness as certain individuals might think. As a matter of fact, according to different sources, there are somewhere in the range of 25 and 26 million diabetics living in the US.

Diabetes isn't simply a sickness that influences more established, overweight individuals; its different kinds can influence newborn children and the older, and in the middle between. To assist with getting a superior handle on the idea of diabetes, it assists with knowing the signs and side effects for different age gatherings. Here are some of them.

Babies Looking for the signs and side effects of diabetes in newborn children can be precarious.

Watch for side effects of low glucose notwithstanding high, caution specialists.

High glucose (hyperglycemia) is generally connected with diabetes, yet low glucose (hypoglycemia) may likewise be a side effect. Infants with low glucose might shake, be testy, or have pale or blue lips or potentially fingers. High glucose might present as lack of hydration, or a child appearing to have to drink constantly and pee habitually. Likewise, a sweetish smell to the pee is demonstrative of diabetes. Different side effects of diabetes in babies incorporate unreasonable languor, outrageous yearning, and wounds that are delayed to mend. A few sources propose searching for a dim rash on the rear of your child's neck, it might feel to some degree smooth. Youngsters Like babies, kids with diabetes might show outrageous thirst and incessant pee. The person might get more fit in spite of all the greedy appetite, and as a matter of fact, a few sources say that unexplained weight reduction is the main indication of diabetes in youngsters. Different side effects include:

Crankiness

Touchiness

Exhaustion Strange way of behaving (simply not behaving like him/herself)

Vision issues, particularly obscured vision that goes back and forth .

Ongoing yeast diseases, particularly in young ladies .

Shivering in hands and feet Grown-ups Grown-ups can foster Sort I or adolescent diabetes, especially youthful grown-ups. Type II diabetes happens sometime down the road and is not the same as Type I, yet the side effects of both are very comparative.

For grown-ups, the accompanying side effects might demonstrate diabetes.

Unexplained weight reduction, Grown-ups specifically should be forewarned about this side effect, since grown-ups frequently think any weight reduction is great.

This is particularly evident assuming their primary care physician let them know that being overweight seriously jeopardized them for diabetes. Yet, in the event that the weight reduction is unexplained and is joined by any of different side effects, it may very well be really smart to see your PCP.

Thirst and pee Like babies and youngsters, grown-ups with undiscovered diabetes are frequently incredibly parched. Furthermore, the more you drink, the more you pee. In the event that it seems as if you just drink and pee, and never feel fulfilled regarding your thirst, diabetes may be the guilty party.

Shivering in limits Similarly as with youngsters, grown-ups may encounter shivering hands and feet.

2.2 In the event that Not Diabetes - What?

There are messes that imitate the side effects of diabetes. Among these are liver sickness, sullen stoutness, and the results of certain cholesterol and pulse bringing down drugs.

2.3 Tips for Preventing Diabetes

Diabetes is a developing issue. Assuming you have diabetes in your family or in any case are in danger, it's a good idea to make a few safeguard strides. Type II diabetes is the most preventable type of the infection. Here are a few hints that might assist with keeping diabetes from creating in your life. Legitimate Eating regimen - Food varieties That Might Forestall Diabetes Many sources recommend that an eating regimen underlining plant food sources is significant for forestalling diabetes. Different food varieties that might assist with balancing out glucose and hold you back from growing all out diabetes incorporate the accompanying:

Magnesium-rich food sources like dark beans, spinach, and almonds are said to assist with forestalling diabetes. Strangely, diabetics are much of the time lacking in magnesium, sources say.

Onions and garlic are normal glucose controllers. Dark bean soup with garlic or dark bean burgers with onions would be perfect!

Stevia is an extremely sweet, calorie free spice; the concentrate is many times sold in supermarkets and wellbeing food stores as a

sugar. It might bring down glucose, as well, pursuing is a decent decision for those with pre-diabetic circumstances or those wishing to forestall the beginning of diabetes.

2.4 Exercise

It's significant for everybody, except for the individuals who wish to forestall diabetes, exercise is particularly fundamental. For a certain something, vivacious action will in general lower glucose.

For another,exercise generally brings about weight reduction assuming it's drilled consistently and appropriately.

Keeping a solid body weight is vital to diabetes counteraction. For good measure. There are a few potential precaution estimates you can take that are dubious, or possibly the jury is still out concerning whether these actions are viable. Assuming they're solid measures, however, it could pay to decide in favor watchfulness and carry out them regardless of whether their viability against diabetes is questionable.

A few instances of this kind of counteraction include:

Lessening pressure, whether through extending, reflection, supplication, or different types of pressure decrease. A few examinations recommend that persistent pressure might build your gamble for creating diabetes.

Decreasing hypertension may likewise assist with forestalling diabetes.

These two circumstances frequently exist together, and research proposes that hypertension might considerably set off the beginning of diabetes. Monitoring your circulatory strain is something sound to do in any case, so you truly can't lose on this one.

High fructose corn syrup, that sugar we as a whole love to detest, might be embroiled in the improvement of diabetes. It very well might be nothing else of an issue than white sugar. Yet again removing HFCS from your eating routine is definitely not something perilous to do and may try to be better, so it's a shared benefit on the off chance that you cut it out of your eating regimen out of the blue.

Trans fats and immersed fats are normally remembered for the "don't eat" list for those wishing to forestall diabetes. It's been proposed that these artery clogging fats can fuel or trigger type II diabetes side effects.

2.5 Living with Diabetes - Pragmatic Advances

Notwithstanding what age you are determined to have diabetes or which of the two sorts you have, it assists with making them adapt methodologies. Living with diabetes can be testing, yet it unquestionably need not hold you down. Here are a few useful strides for living with diabetes. Interfacing with Others Perhaps the most supportive thing you can do is become a piece of the diabetes local area in your space. You'll learn you're in good company; you'll presumably get important data, tips, and writing, and you'll find out about impending occasions, withdrawals, and camps. This can be useful for youngsters who need to find a place with a friend but doesn't know how or then again in the event that others will acknowledge them, or for grown-ups who feel confined in their condition. It helps a ton just to realize there are other people who comprehend what it's like.

Have a group

On the off chance that you don't have a neighborhood support bunch for diabetics, consider framing one.

 Individuals can meet at your home or at a neighborhood scene, and you can set up person to person communication or a site to stay in contact. You would design excursions, get-togethers, gatherings, etc, and keep your gathering informed about occasions.

Take Control

While standard visits to your doctor are significant, diabetics eventually must be answerable for their own day to day care. You need to figure out how to take your own glucose and control your own insulin, and just know when something feels "off." It depends on you to carry out an activity routine and eat the right food varieties. Realizing this essential truth, you are answerable for dealing with your diabetes, you can remove a portion of the pressure from living with this condition. Try not to Whip Yourself For those with Type II diabetes or for guardians of kids who have Type I, it tends to be enticing to become involved with oneself attempting finger pointing. The improvement of Type II diabetes may as a matter of fact be connected to specific way of life decisions, yet it's not really so; and regardless of whether it is, you need to push ahead and into a sound way of life. Guardians whose youngsters or kids have Type I might fault themselves, moms might stress over something they did while pregnant, or fixate on allowing their kid to eat a great deal of sugar before the conclusion. These faults are not really fundamentally even obvious! It sits around idly to stress, so center around pushing ahead and capitalizing on life from now on. This might be the start of a chance for personal development and self control.

Have a plan

Having an arrangement can assist you with remaining in charge in a given circumstance, and capitalize on gatherings and occasions. Choose quite a bit early the way in which you will deal with occasion and party treats so you don't need to think and react quickly each time you're offered a treat.

Chapter 3 Treatment for Diabetes

There are generally a lot of examinations happening in the field of diabetes. Researchers are continuously searching for a fix or better treatment, growing new medications and gear, and performing different things with immature microorganisms and different techniques.

New treatment choices are opening up constantly.

As a diabetic, keeping your glucose levels consistent is critical. When you have that taken care of, numerous diabetics like to look through elective medicines. Related to your doctor's information, you might find your wellbeing is upgraded by at least one elective medicine.

We should investigate a portion of the treatment choices accessible for diabetics. Insulin Those with Type I diabetes should accept insulin. This should be possible as a shot, which the diabetic gives oneself (with the exception of little kids, whose guardians could offer the day to day chances). Another choice is an insulin siphon, which is outside the body however connected by a little cylinder. The diabetic enters what the person in question eats into the siphon, and the siphon creates the fundamental insulin. For Type II diabetics, insulin could possibly be fundamental. Assuming that it is, there are a few distinct choices for these diabetics. Breathed in or even oral insulin might be recommended, or customary shots or "pens."

3.1 Prescriptions

Notwithstanding insulin, a few diabetics take different prescriptions. A few meds, similar to Metformin, work by diminishing the glucose that the liver produces, which supports the body's reaction to insulin. Others, like Glipizide and Glimepiride, increment the pancreas' own insulin. This, obviously, brings down glucose; yet probably it would possibly be successful assuming the pancreas actually worked fairly. Some fresher meds are called DPP4 inhibitors. These influence the pancreas both by invigorating the emission of insulin and by decreasing the discharge of a chemical called glucagon. Glucagon raises glucose.

3.2 Options

A few normal substances have been considered for their capacity to lower or settle glucose. Chromium, a mineral that happens normally in the entire sugar stick, might be low in individuals with Type II diabetes. Chromium is said to settle glucose. Different minerals, spices, and food sources that are said to assist with glucose are:

Stevia

Magnesium (diabetics are in many cases viewed as lacking in this mineral)

Fundamental unsaturated fats Cinnamon

Ginseng Needle therapy has likewise been investigated as an elective treatment for diabetes. Diet and exercise are significant for all diabetics, however these basics are typically thought of as "elective medicines," most likely in light of the fact that they don't straightforwardly include drugs or customary treatment. In any case, exercise and diet are significant for keeping glucose managed and keeping a solid body weight.

Chapter 4 :Managing Diabetes with Diet and Exercise - Top Tips

Type II diabetes, as a rule, is the rendition of this infection that can be made do with diet and exercise. Nonetheless, for those with Type I, these sound way of life tips might assist with letting side effects and upgrade the executives free from the condition. Here are a few ways to oversee diabetes with diet and exercise. The Right Carbs, or sugars, have been on the "terrible" list of late. However, much the same as fat, there are great and awful carbs, particularly with regards to diabetes, the executives. By and large, to keep away from could incorporate the accompanying:

White sugar

White flour

White rice

Natural product juices

Degermed cornmeal Carbs to underscore could incorporate these food varieties:

Entire organic products

Entire grains

Earthy colored rice

Entire cornmeal Proteins and Carbs Joining proteins and carbs at dinners and bites can assist with forestalling glucose spikes. Models include: Entire grain bread with unsweetened nut spread.

Entire grain wafers with low-fat cheddar
Lean turkey bosom in an entire wheat pita
Earthy colored rice and beans
"Party blend" produced using entire grain cereal, peanuts, and pretzels
Apple cuts with peanut butter
Earthy colored rice and seared salmon
Entire wheat macaroni and cheddar (made with low-fat cheddar and skim milk) Fats While keeping your weight at a sound level is significant for dealing with your diabetes, eating the right sort of fat has its place. With some restraint, these solid fats can assist with bringing down cholesterol and give other medical advantages.
Sound fats can be viewed as in:
Fish (particularly salmon and Cold singe)
Avocados
Almonds
Olive, safflower, and canola oils It's smart to keep away from soaked fats and trans fats (hydrogenated fats). Soaked fats will be fats like spread and shortening that are strong at room temperature. Hydrogenated fats were once fluid fats (some of the time sound ones) that were misleadingly set utilizing hydrogen. Trans or hydrogenated fats are tracked down in certain sorts of peanut butter and in margarine, and in

the fixing arrangements of endless bundled food sources.

4.1 Exercise

To deal with your diabetes exercise is considered by specialists to be fundamental. Curiously, strength preparing has been demonstrated to be particularly useful to diabetics, delivering results that, in certain cases, rival prescription. Oxygen consuming activity is additionally useful; it gets the pulse up and consumes calories. The significant thing is to exercise no less than 30 minutes per day for at least five days per week. This helps hold your weight under control (essential for diabetics and pre-diabetics) and may try to lessen pressure. Stress has been ensnared.